The Magic of Basil – *Tulsi*

To Heal Naturally

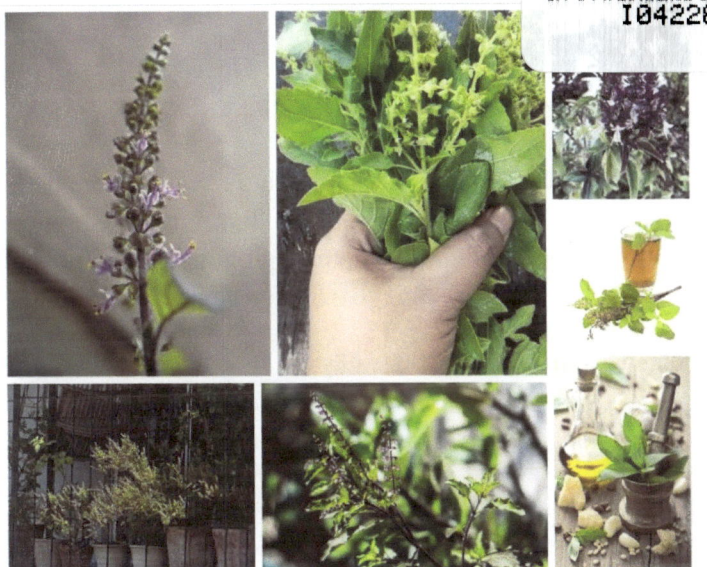

Dueep Jyot Singh

Natural Remedy Series

Mendon Cottage Books

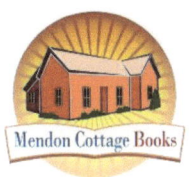

JD-Biz Publishing

Our books are available at

1. Amazon.com
2. Barnes and Noble
3. Itunes
4. Kobo
5. Smashwords
6. Google Play Books

Table of Contents

Introduction

Basil has long been known as a valuable herb through the ages, when it was used to flavor foods. But this herb has also been a valuable an integral part of ancient alternative medicine. More than 4000 years ago, one of the greatest of ancient doctors Charaka wrote in his compendium that the juice from the leaves of the sacred basil mixed with honey taken three times a day could cure patients suffering from whooping cough and chest ailments.

That was the time when people relied on natural cures, and their own inmate good health to keep healthy and live long. I am proud to present this book to you, about one of the most useful herbs available to mankind today, of which the significant benefits have been written in ancient books of the East.

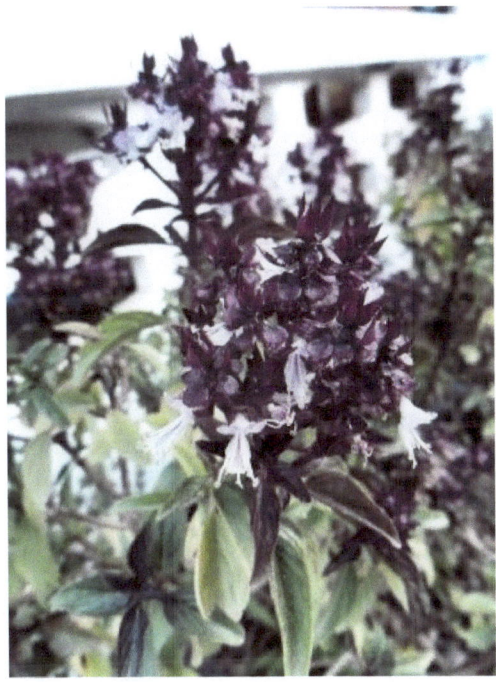

Oscimum sanctum is the scientific name given to the sacred basil. What is the difference between cooking basil and sacred basil? Well, to tell you very frankly, most of the cooks in the East prefer to use the plant, which has purplish colored leaves, in their food, just before serving. They call that the cooking basil. On the other hand, the sacred basil has smaller and greener leaves, more pungent in odor and in taste.

One rule passed down from the ancients is that milk and Basil do not mix. So when you are getting rid of a cough and cold, you make up a mixture of one teaspoonful each of honey and dried ginger, eight black peppercorns, and 5 to 10 basil leaves and boil them in water. Drink them down twice a day, and there goes your cold. But if you are boiling these ingredients in milk, leave the basil leaves out.

Sacred basil has a religious and mythological significance coming down the ages, both in the East and in the West. The Greek Eastern Orthodox church used basil in traditional rituals and the women of the house used to sprinkle sacred basil on the threshold of their houses on St. Basil's day celebrated on 1 January in order to usher in a new and fruitful prosperous new year.

In almost every Hindu household, in India the garden has to have a sacred basil plant. It is called Tulsi –[tool-see]. This plant is grown on a platform, which is easily accessible from all four corners of the house. It is decorated with religious and mythological images of gods and goddesses, and then the plant is planted on top of the pillar. Every morning, Hindu women have a bath, light a lamp and then water the Tulsi in their house. The women bow to it in obeisance, because they are wishing the goddess Tulsi welcome to their house this day. They are also praying for the well-being of their family for the day, with the blessings of the goddess.

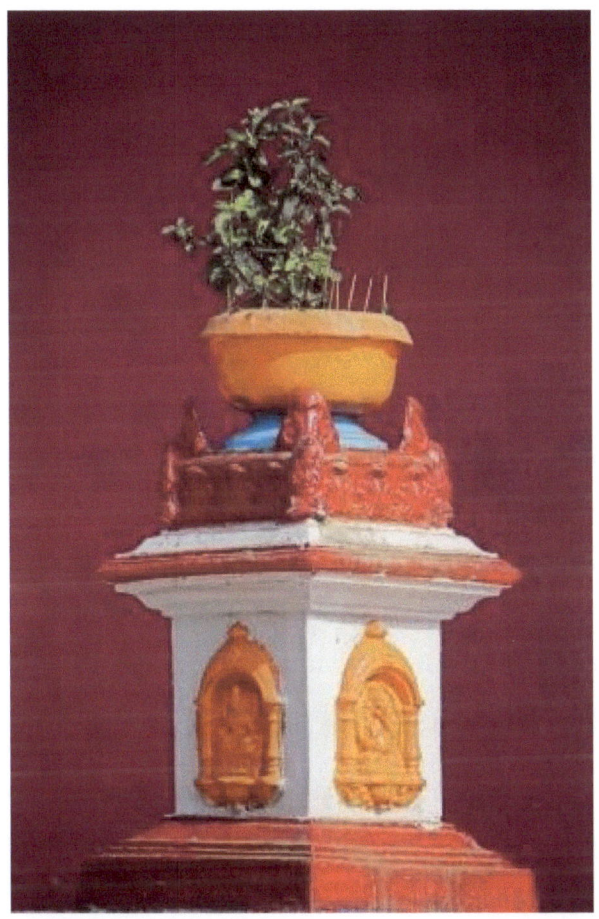

In Hindu mythology, Tulsi , also known as Vrinda was the consort of Lord Krishna. That is why the place where she dwells is called Vrindavana-the garden/forest of Vrinda. The platform in which a Tulsi is planted is thus called Vrindavana.

In ancient times, they used to place a lit lamp in front of this plant at sunset. This tradition is still followed in Orthodox and traditional households to this day.

In ancient times, man had to fall back on natural resources in order to keep healthy. The ancients knew the value of some of these plants, so they decided that the best way to make the common person treasure, trust and use it was to make it a part of religious and symbolical rituals. This is what is done to many trees and herbs in the East. So even if one does not follow the religious ritualism, one can always bless these plants for their usefulness and for their benefit to mankind in general.

I am not a Hindu. But having lived all over India for a major part of my life, I immediately recognize the mythological and powerful significance, this plant had in the lives of the Hindus. I used to treat this plant as an herb use for cooking and curing diseases. They revere it as a sacred manifestation of the gods. After all, it is considered to be the panacea of all ills, and any house with a Tulsi plant growing in it is never going to suffer from disease, sickness and bad luck, that is the belief passed down from the ancients.

Just like the neem tree, the Tulsi is also considered to be a wonderful air purifier. As they say, familiarity breeds contempt. That is why, when you are in the presence of a plant, which is growing so commonly in the East, you do not bother much about its medical and religious and culinary significance. Unfortunately, that is what has happened to this plant in the East of today. It is grown in the gardens, just because your neighbor handed you one of the saplings and you had an empty pot handy.

But you are going to get to know more about the versatile uses this plant can be put, to give you a continuous long life and a healthy one.

The use of Tulsi in naturopathy , thanks to ancient treatises has now been proven scientifically, because researchers have found out that this plant has strong antifungal, antiviral and antibacterial properties.

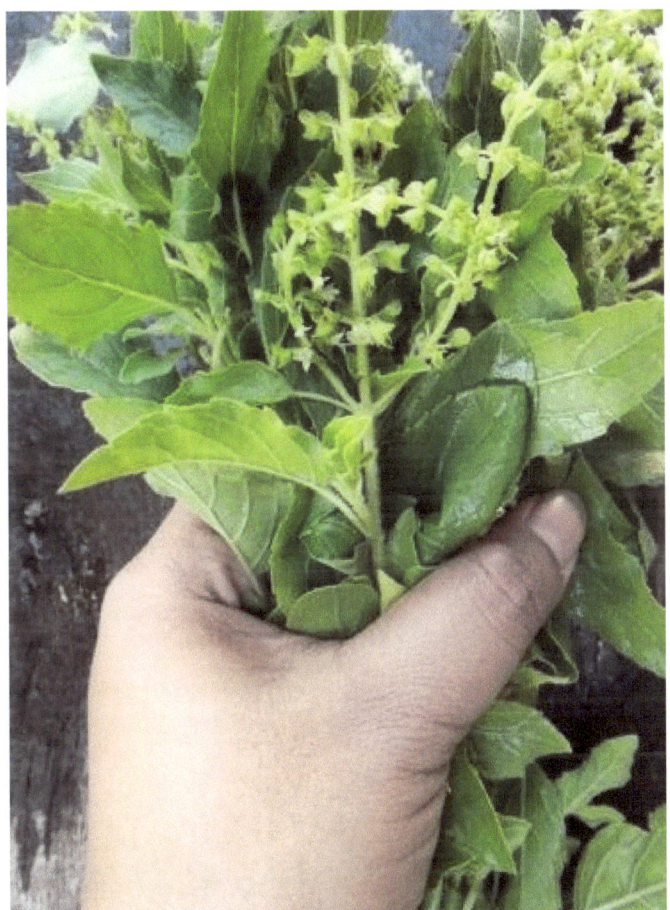

That is why many of the diseases which are caused by fungii, bacteria, and viruses can be cured or even prevented with the leaves of this plant.

In many parts of the East, it is a natural automatic gesture to eat five leaves, fresh off the plant, before one leaves for the office or starts the daily grind. Not only does this keep the breath sweet, but it also keeps your body toned and healthy.

Tulsi is considered to be a preventative as well as a curative. So if you want to meditate in the open air you would want to sit down in front of a neem tree, or a Tulsi plant, where you can breathe fresh pure oxygen.

I was looking through many ancient herb books, written by writers in the East and the West. I noticed that many of them spoke about gathering those herbs on a particular day, under a particular moon, or while undergoing some particular ritual. Being of a scientific turn of mind, I understood the motive behind all this ritualism. This would enforce and auto suggest the power of that particular herb in the minds of the users, when compared to herbs gathered, just by walking into your herb garden and plucking them off the branches and shoots.

Tulsi does not have any particular ritual for gathering the leaves, seeds, and flowers, as far as I know. But because it has become a part of tradition and religious symbolism, it is thus valued in the households where it is worshiped.

The value of basil is not underestimated in the West either. John Keats's poem The Pot of Basil in which the tragic Isabella "hung over her sweet Basil evermore,/And moistened it with tears unto the core."

http://en.wikipedia.org/wiki/Isabella_and_the_Pot_of_Basil

William H. Hunt painted a scene from this poem using the features of his dead wife for Isabella's portrait. The reason why the ladies treasured this plan so much, was because she had buried the head of her murdered love, Lorenzo in it. Taking this poem not in its literally aspect, but in its significant aspect, one goes back to medieval times in Italy when herbs like basil were extremely precious and held sacred. So that is why she honored the being most precious to her by planting his head in an equally priceless plant.

This does sound rather gruesome to our modern and more sensitive sensibilities, but that was what life was like in the Middle Ages.

How to Grow Basil

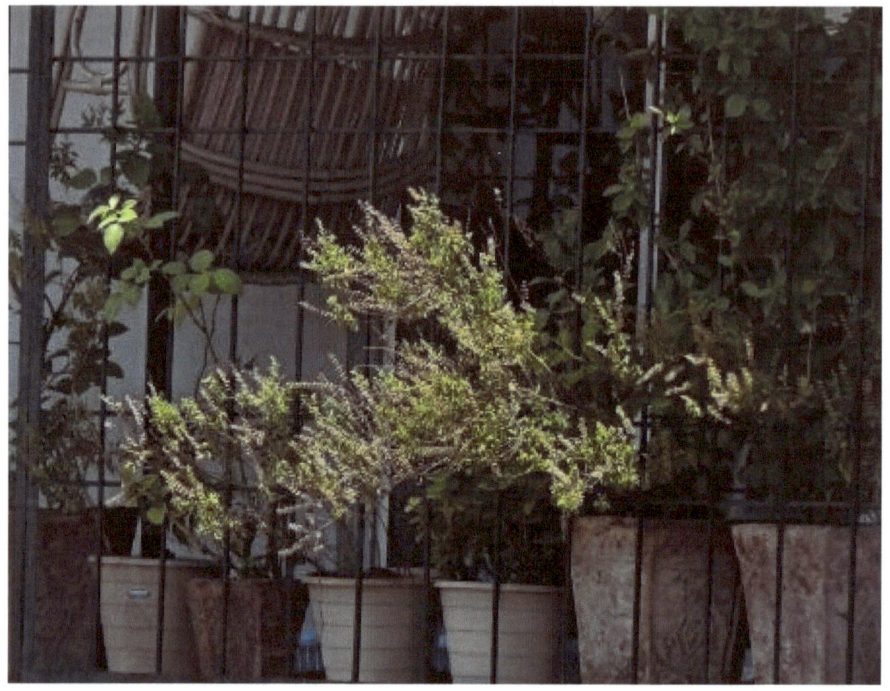

The Tulsi can be grown very easily in Clay pots. It needs steady watering every day. Otherwise it is going to start dwindling away. Again, the religious significance – pour water into the plant every morning, if and when you worship it. The ancients knew all about human psychology, and also about how to get them to utilize these beneficial herbs.

A normal Tulsi plant is going to be about three – 4 feet high, when fully grown. It can grow in any type of soil. However, the best soil for it is Clay and well moisturized well fertilized soil. You should have an excellent drainage system. Just sprinkle the seeds gathered off another plant, in your prepared area, cover with a layer of soil, and keep watering. They are going to sprout within a couple of days.

You can then transplant the sprouts to other parts of your garden or leave the ones which seem the most healthy in your pots. There are two types of Basil – one has black branches and purplish green leaves. The other has white branches and light green/dark green leaves. Both of them are equal in beneficial power and potency. Nevertheless, the one with white branches is considered to be better for herbal remedies, because it is stronger, while the one with black branches is excellent for using in cooking.

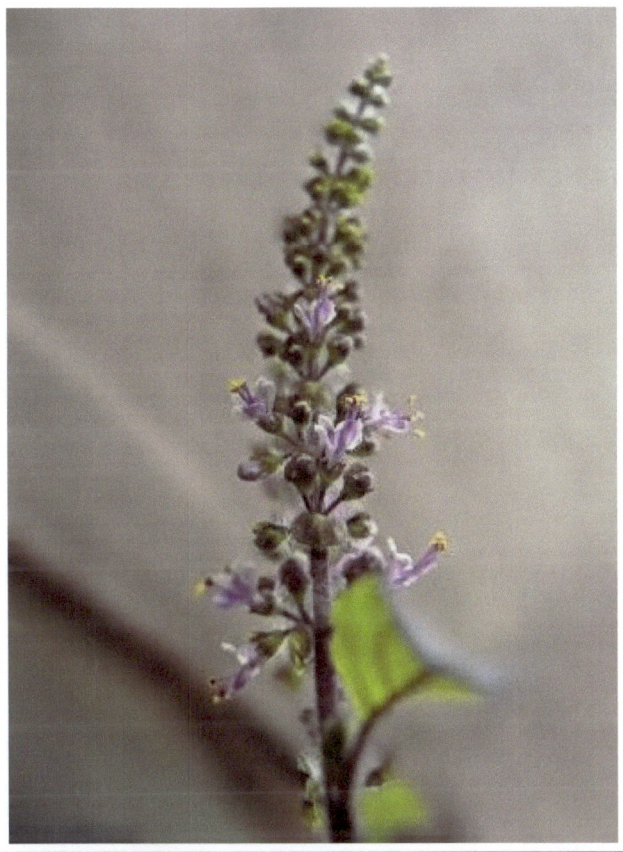

Powdered Basil As a Herb

The powdered basil which you buy from the market is the dried and ground leaves of the cooking basil. You sun dry them by collecting the leaves early in the morning, placing them on a cloth, and folding the cloth so that they do not get dusty. Then place them in the shade and allow to dry for 4 to 5 days. These leaves are now ready for grinding and using in your cuisine as a spice and Herb.

Basil loses its flavor, if you fry it with other herbs. So I would recommend that you just sprinkle basil after the dish has been cooked and mix thoroughly. This is going to give the dish a delicious smelling aroma.

Basil is called Rehan in Israel, Georgia, Turkey and Arihani in Swahili. In Spanish, you are going to ask for Arrayan when you want Basil.

Getting rid of Malarial Fever

This was told to me by a naturopath doctor in the mountains. Ever since Quinine and cinchona was discovered as the best way in which you could cure malarial fevers, it has been used extensively to lower the temperature and to cure the patient. However, the patient is not going to be told about the side effects of cinchona. Prolonged use can cause toxic complications.

You may suffer from headache and excess of sweating. Along with that, you need to drink this with milk and orange juice to neutralize the hot "nature" of cinchona.

Most of the people in the East still cannot afford orange juice to heal themselves. So they went back to ancient remedies which were not so complicated. This was mixing six peppercorns and 4 leaves of Tulsi in a glass full of water, and then boiling until the water was reduced to half its quantity. This was fed to the patient twice a day until the fever disappeared and the patient was cured.

You can also feed the patient 2 tablespoons of fresh Tulsi leaves juice twice a day along with honey. Anybody suffering from periodic bouts of malaria could prevent this from occurring by eating five leaves of fresh Tulsi morning and evening, all throughout the winter and autumn.

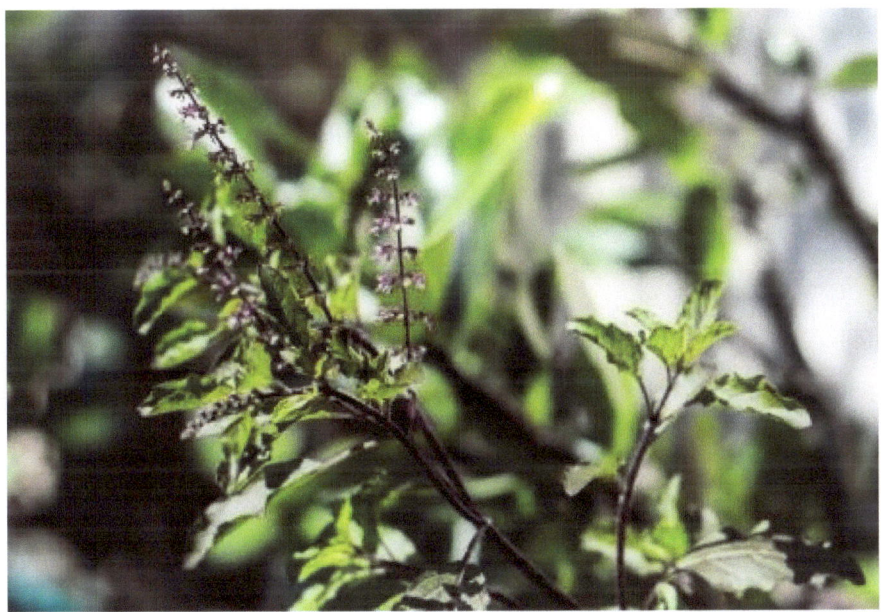

A British botanist Sir George Woodward got this "Mosquito Plant" and planted it in the Victoria Gardens and Albert Museum in Mumbai. To his great surprise, the mosquitoes disappeared like bad nightmares. That means that the fear of malaria was also lessened considerably in those insalubrious seaside areas, especially during the dreaded Indian monsoon.

This was an experiment done by some researchers some years ago. They tried this experiment on rats by feeding them Tulsi leaves and injecting them with potentially lethal carbon tetrachloride. The rats survived without any damage to their livers.

Fever in the Winter

Try this remedy too, if you are suffering from fever in the winter. Make up a mixture of black pepper – three peppercorns is enough. I feel with 2 tablespoons molasses and Tulsi leaves. Put them in a glass of water, and allow to boil until you have half the amount. Then add half a teaspoonful of lemon juice. Drink this piping hot every three hours. This is great for getting rid of any sort of fever in the winter. All you have to do is cover yourself up with a blanket and go to sleep and wait for the black pepper and Tulsi induced sweat to get rid of the germs, the infection, and the high-temperature.

If you do not want to take this boiling mixture, you can take 10 g of Tulsi juice, with 1 g pepper powder – one peppercorn – and 1 teaspoon of honey. Feed this to the patient and watch the flavor go down.

In the same way, you can take one teaspoonful of ginger juice and 2 teaspoons of Tulsi juice once every day to rid yourself of fever.

Influenza

Take 50 g of fresh Tulsi leaves. Add five peppercorns to them, and mix thoroughly. Now put them in 200 g of boiling hot water, and allow to reduce to half its amount. Finish these hundred grams in three doses throughout the day.

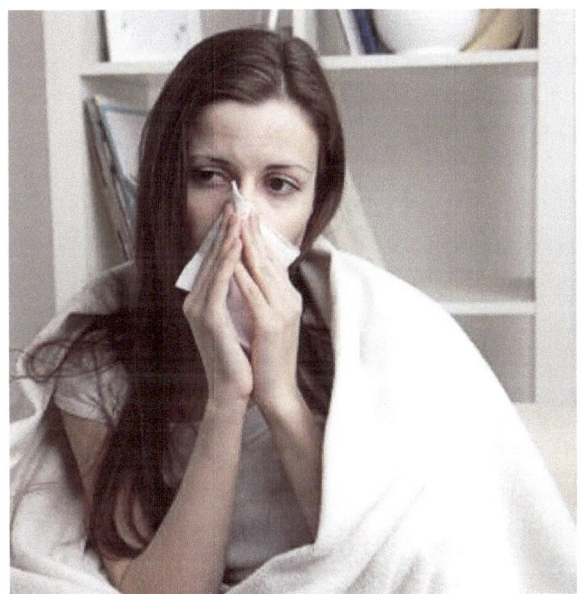

If you do not want to go through the process of boiling them, so 25 g of Tulsi leaves in 250 g of hot water. Now, grind them. Drink hundred grams of this water mixed with another hundred grams of hot water three times a day.

Rock Salt Cure

You can also try this rock salt cure. Take 10 g of Tulsi leaves in 150 g of water, allow to boil till about 50 g is left. Filter and add rock salt to taste. Sip this slowly and when it is still warm once a day.

If you do not have rock salt around, you can try this same remedy by adding ordinary sugar in 10 g juice, in one cup of water and boiled for a couple of minutes. Our job is to take the full benefit of the powerful aromatic essential oils in basil.

Preventive and Curative Fever Cures in Winter

You can try this remedy both to prevent as well as cure fevers, brought about by winter, and exposure to the harsh elements. Take 5 g – 1 teaspoon each of two fee leaves, ginger and mint leaves, put them in one glass of water and boil till they are half the amount. Drink it down, once a day, if you are not suffering from fever and twice a day, if you are suffering from fever!

A Basil Sanatorium

This was an idea suggested by a person in an area where people suffered a lot from chest infections, including TB and other lung related problems. He asked the people of that area to make a Basil sanatorium.

This was done by taking a little bit of land and sowing Basil extensively over it. In between these plants, he suggested erecting huts made out of bamboo and mud. After all, this was the natural sanatorium for healing those people who could not afford to go to the mountains to Sanatoriums and get cured of potentially fatal diseases.

The patients could live in such healthy air, and take full advantage of the aromatic healing oil of the basil. This could strengthen their lungs and improve their circulatory system. Along with that, they could take the leaves of Tulsi along with other healthy natural products like honey under the supervision of a good doctor and get cured.

Did you know that in Eastern cuisine food is still tempered with oil, and spices as it has been done for millenniums? But in ancient times, the juice from the Tulsi leaves was extracted, and tempering of food was done in this juice extract.

Ginger Tulsi Tea

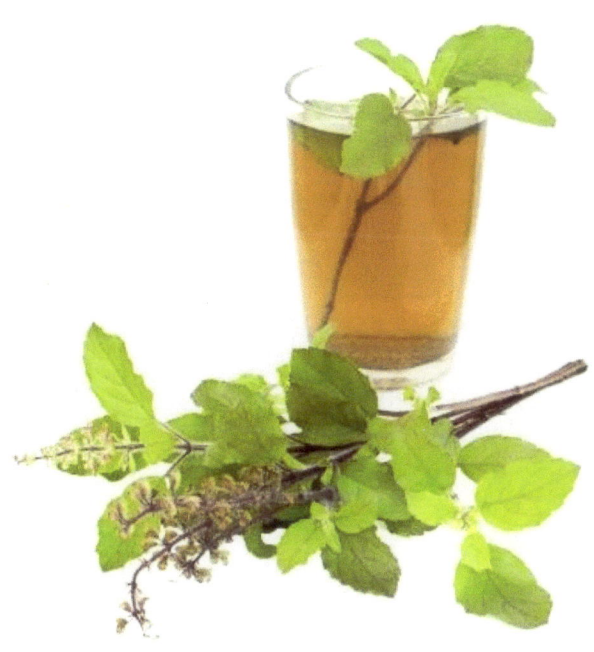

This is something which every person getting ready for a harsh winter notes down as something to be drunk at least once every day. You are going to make a mixture of one teaspoonful of Tulsi leaves, and 10 g of either grated raw ginger or one teaspoonful of dried ginger powder and make a ginger tea. When it is boiling, add hot milk and honey or sugar to taste. This is going to keep you healthy throughout the winter. This is normally drunk with the accompaniment of tea masala which is a mixture of spices like cloves, cardamoms and cinnamon. You just need a pinch of these spices in this tea to keep you warm and healthy throughout the cold winter.

Mint Tea for Slimming

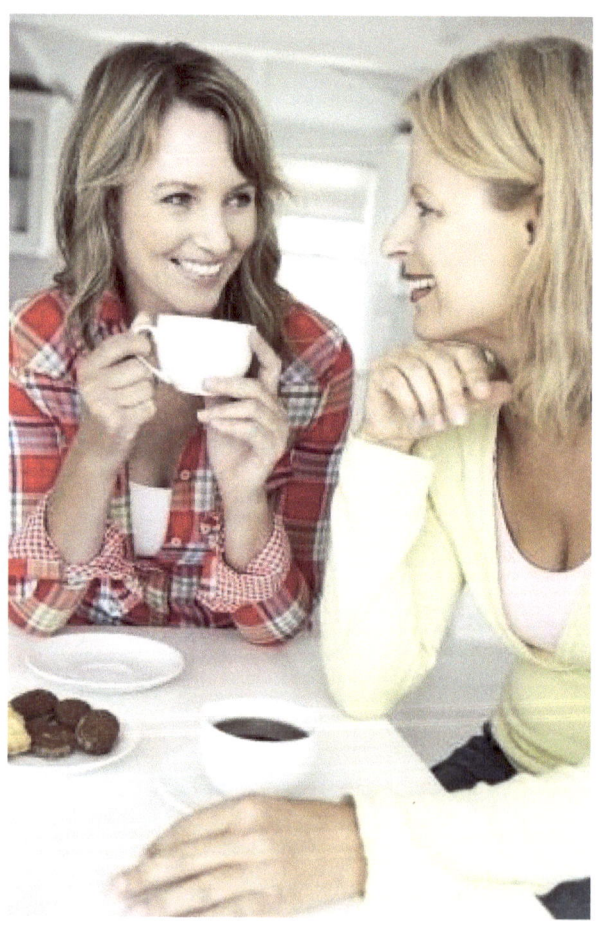

You can also try out this version of a healthy tea, with 12 leaves of Tulsi, two pieces of lemongrass and 12 leaves of mint. Boil for 15 minutes and then filter. You can now add honey and lemon juice to taste. Drink this every morning on an empty stomach. This is considered to be a good drink for slimming. You can also add a little bit of ginger.

Suffering from Acidity?

Try mixing some fresh or powdered leaves of basil to yogurt. Eat this every day until you find yourself cured. I normally add some rock salt and pepper, just for taste, but I know that I am going be cured by the basil.

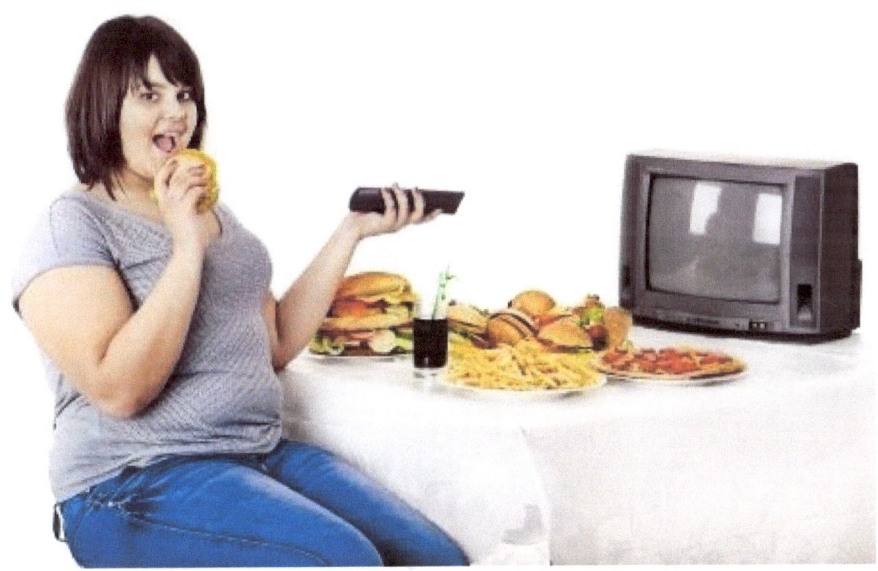

Overeating junk food WILL cause acidity.

This is something which women readers will find rather chauvinistic, but my medical encyclopedia of information told me that this was due to their different biophysiological and chemical makeup, along with their own female hormones. Women need to drink basil when they are curing themselves, with yogurt or buttermilk. That is because these leaves are extremely hot in nature.

So if you want a refreshing drink in the winter, just mix up three crushed basil leaves in a glass of buttermilk or a spoonful of yogurt.

Men can get away with a warming drink of hot water with one spoon full of molasses, five, crushed leaves of Tulsi and one spoon full of lemon juice in the winter. Do not drink this in the summer.

Just a tip – if you are heating to see juice, do not use honey. Honey should never be taken after it has been heated because all its power has disappeared by then. Nevertheless, hot milk and honey is the only exception here, used to cure insomnia.

Who Should Not Take Basil?

According to Ayurveda, people suffering from hemorrhoids and piles should never use basil and pepper. In the same way, if you are drinking milk, avoid garlic, onions, carrots, Tulsi, radishes, meat, and molasses in the same meal. However, you can take these products with yogurt.

How to Use Basil for Natural Remedies

Five – 25 leaves are enough for children. Adults can take more in the winter, and less in the summer. That can be anywhere between 25 – hundred leaves. Grind the leaves with a little bit of water and drink 4 to 10 g, depending on the ailment. 1 teaspoon is 6 g.

Eat or drink this juice or chew the leaves first thing in the morning on an empty stomach.

Caffeine addiction?

If you are suffering from a caffeine addiction, try drinking a brew made up of Tulsi leaves. This will slowly and steadily cure you of that "coffee hit" before you find yourself mentally and physically prepared for the day's work.

Tulsi for beauty

I have already spoken about meditating in a place where there is a Tulsi around. That is good to keep your system fresh and going. In the same manner, you can keep your skin beautiful and refreshed by making a Tulsi facemask.

Grind five dry leaves of the Tulsi and use this powder to exfoliate your skin. Not only is this going to get rid of all the dead cells and the grime, but it is also going to get rid of any potential blemishes and skin diseases on your body.

Using the Tulsi Steamer

Add some hot water to your steamer. Put half a teaspoonful of lemon juice in it along with a fistful each of mint and Tulsi leaves. Bring to a boil, cover your face with a towel and allow your skin to steam in this fragrant aromatic luxuriant steam. When the water gets lukewarm, you can wash your whole body with it to get that refreshing minty tingle. This is an excellent natural deodorizer too. You can bottle up the liquid when it is cold, and use it to wash the sweaty portions of your body to keep the skin fresh.

Dark Patches

If you have dark patches on your skin, do not despair. Just extract the juice of some Tulsi leaves and add a little bit of lemon juice to it. Apply it all over the dark patches and wait for the paste to get dry. I normally apply the leaves along with the juice to my skin. Wash it off with lukewarm water. Do this two times, every day until you find those dark patches disappearing.

If you do not have lemon juice around, you can use a little bit of ginger juice. 10 to 15 drops- not more than that because ginger is more powerful than lemon juice.

Whooping cough/dry Cough

Do you have somebody in the family suffering from whooping cough or even dry cough? Just take 1 teaspoon each of grated fresh green leaves of the Tulsi, and ginger and add them to one teaspoonful of honey. Give this once a day until the patient is cured completely due to the antiseptic properties of honey and basil.

Traditional Cough Syrup

This is the traditional cough syrup still being used in areas, where people do not have access to modern sources of medicine, or they find them too expensive.

Take 5 g each of Tulsi leaves juice, bishops weed, and turmeric. Blend them together. Now add 25 g of honey to this mixture, and bottle in a glass bottle. Give children half a teaspoonful – 30 – 50 drops of this syrup twice or thrice a day. You can have one teaspoonful, because you are an adult.

This is another remedy given to me by a friend, who believes greatly in the beneficial properties of Tulsi, and keeps on experimenting. She used to add 4 to 5 leaves of Tulsi to the ordinary tea that she boiled every morning and evening. Once her kiddie came down with a cold, and she gave him 2 tablespoons of that tea – yes, boiled with tea leaves and with milk and sugar – twice a day. She says that he was cured within 2 to 3 days. She now swears by this remedy as an excellent cold/cough remedy. I told her that the brewing process in itself was enough to dilute the power of the leaves, but yet mild enough to cure a three-year-old kid.

Surefire Cold Remedy Powder

I normally make this in the beginning of winter, so that I do not have to worry about collecting all the ingredients, when I may possibly suffer from cold or influenza. That is when I want to drink something warm, get into bed, and hibernate like the rest of the Bears.

So when you have the time, get together 25 g each of ginger powder, black pepper, molasses/Jaggery and basil leaves. Powder them together and put them in a glass jar. The moment you feel a cold or fever coming on, just take half a teaspoonful of this very powerful powder, and boil it in one glass of water. When you have about a cup, drink this down, while still bearably hot. Drink this twice a day. No fever, no cough, no cold.

Fever Prevention in Children

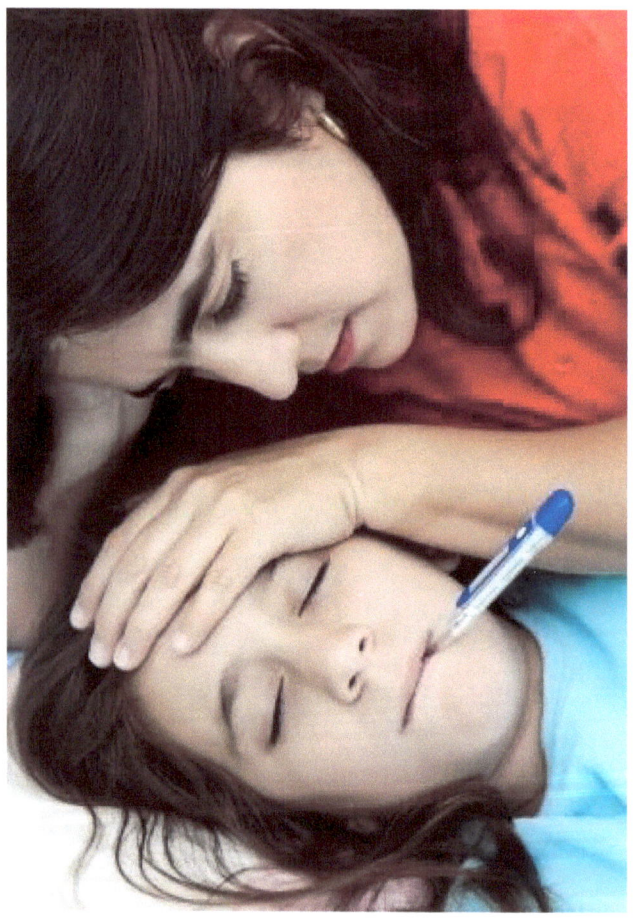

This is a remedy which has been in use since ancient times, to prevent common childhood ailments and fever in children. This can be done by taking 2 g of Tulsi seeds and feeding your kids that every day. You can also supplementing this healthy preventative by giving them the juice of two leaves warmed up slightly on a teaspoon.

Suffering from Chronic Cough?

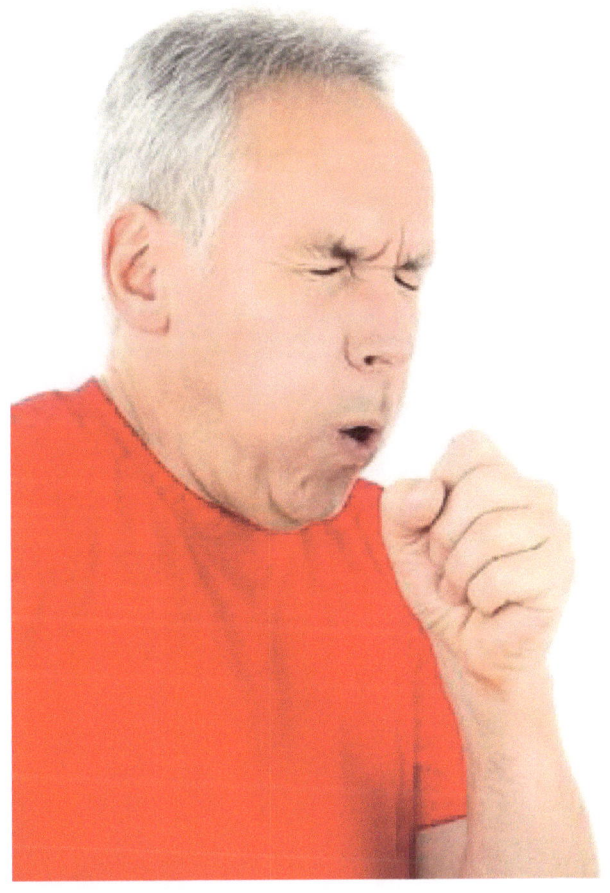

Now this is a time tested remedy. Take seven leaves of the black basil – the leaves are going to be purple in color, and you normally use them for cooking. Take five peppercorns, and mix them together. Make small pellets and put them in a glass bottle. Take one pellet three times a day with water for just one week. Believe it or not, this is the best remedy for chronic cough.

Curing Eczema

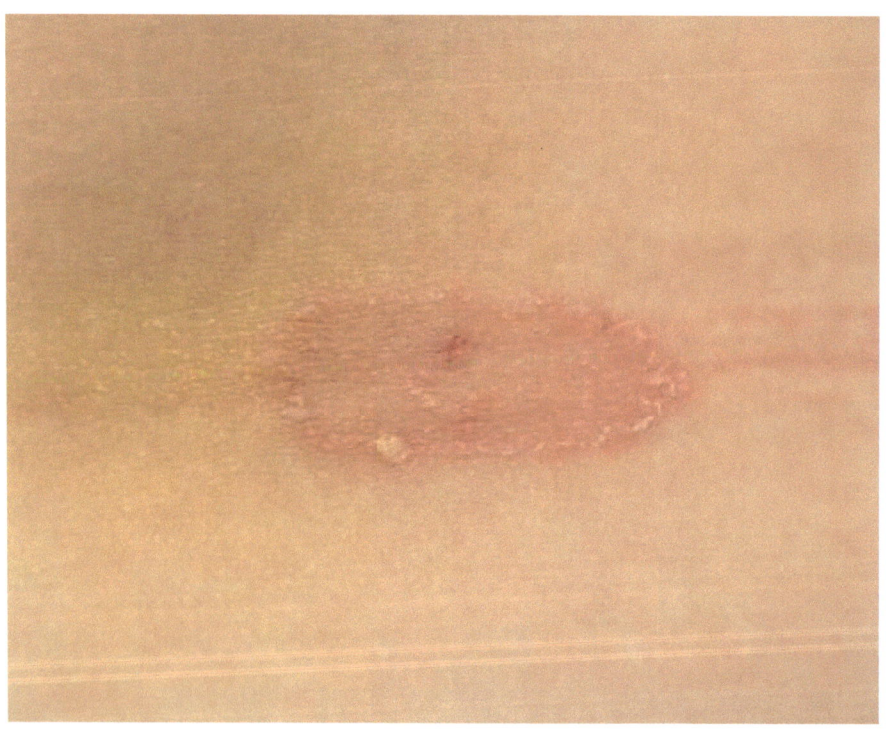

Grind six leaves of Tulsi with half a teaspoonful of lemon juice. Apply this on the affected areas until the eczema is cured completely.

In the same manner, you can get rid of plenty of skin diseases, by making a paste of basil leaves and neem leaves, and applying the paste all over the affected skin areas.

Skin Oil

This is one massage/skin oil, given to me by an herbalist. She said that it would cure any problems on my skin, while keeping it supple and well moisturized.

Take some Tulsi leaves and burn them in, mustard oil. When they are cooked, allow to cool and filter the oil. Apply this all over your skin, which has been affected by any sort of skin ailments. Mustard oil smells, so you can try the same in coconut oil. The moisturizing effect is equally effective, but mustard oil is unrefined and stronger and more powerful.

To Cure Wounds

Make this a part of your herbal medicine closet. Dry two fistfuls of Tulsi leaves in the shade. Now add 1 tablespoon full of powdered alum to this mixture, grind to a fine powder and filter. Place them in a glass bottle. The next time somebody suffers from a cut or a wound, or you have to do is sprinkle this powder on that mixture, and allow the Tulsi to cure the injured tissue naturally.

You can also do this with a mixture of powdered leaves and powdered camphor. Whatever you find easy to use and easily available.

I got rid of an infection of a cut which had been neglected by washing the area in a decoction of boiled basil leaves and then sprinkling dry leaves on that affected area, and bandaging it. This got rid of all the infectious material in the scabs while preventing it from turning into water filled "bubbles." Keep renewing every day, with fresh washing of the wounds, and sprinkling with dry basil leaves until completely cured.

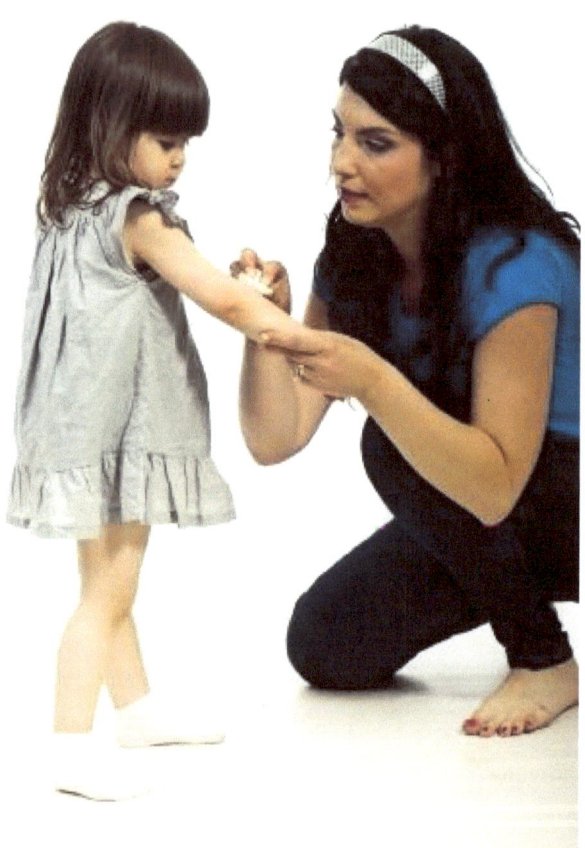

Curing Burns

If the Burns are not very serious, and do not need immediate hospitalization I would suggest that you just make up a mixture of fresh basil leaves juice in coconut oil, and applying it all over the area. This is going to prevent wounds, infections and

Basil in Cuisine

Basil is normally used in stuffing poultry and turkey, especially for the Thanksgiving feast, along with other herbs, like Rosemary, thyme and sage. So, before I give you some recipes, in which you can use basil, here is an easy way, through which you can preserve basil in winter.

Preserving Basil Leaves

Collect the basil leaves in the summer, because that is the time when they are going to give you the best growth of fresh leaves. You can either drive them, but it is better to keep them fresh and green. That can be done by removing all the leaves spreading them on a tray, and placing them in your freezer.

When they have frozen, – in about an hour – put them into an airtight plastic zip lock bag and place them back into your freezer. The same thing can also be done with other herbs, like parsley. In this manner, you can have fresh herbs and leaves ready at hand during the cold winter.

Basil Pesto – a Genoese Dish

It is going to take 15 minutes for preparing this pesto-paste- for 4 hungry people.

One huge bouquet of cooking basil.
25 g pine nuts. You can also use any other nuts you like. Macadamia is also good.
70 g Parmesan cheese, grated, are any other Italian cheese, like Pecorino
Two cloves of garlic, crushed

5 tablespoons olive oil

Salt and pepper to taste

Take 2 tablespoons olive oil in your frying pan, or Wok and gently fry the pine nuts on low heat until they are golden. Allow to cool. When it is cool, add the garlic stir the nuts, and blend in a mixer.

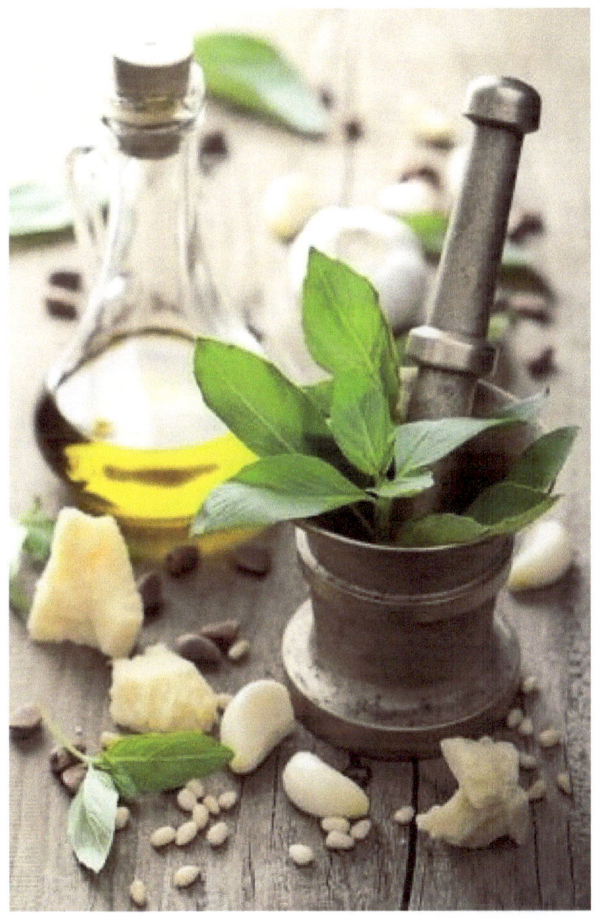

Dry the basil after washing thoroughly and add to the pine mixture in the blender. Also add the cheese and the rest of the olive oil, and blend to get a coarse puree. Add seasonings as necessary, according to taste. Grind again and serve as an accompaniment to snacks. You can also refrigerate it. I use this as a sauce over pasta and macaroni. Delicious. Also try adding a fistful of mint leaves when you are making the pesto. That is another contrasting flavor.

Healthy Sprouts Mix

Try this chutney, with your meals. This is extremely healthy, because it is made up of **20 g sprouted mung and 10 g each of sprouted chickpeas and fenugreek.** To this, add **5 g of peanuts seeds and 10 g each of mint and green coriander.**

Then take **5 g each of ginger, Tulsi leaves, molasses, – dates for diabetics – rock salt and garlic.**

Mix them all together and add one days spoonful of lemon juice to it, along with **15 g coconut water.**

This is an extremely delicious chutney, which is rich in potassium, protein, calcium, sulfur, and also really good Digestive enzymes. This is recommended for people suffering from lethargy, acidity, constipation, and even diabetes.

Conclusion

I have not managed to touch 1/8th of the uses to which you can put basil. But make it an integral part of your kitchen garden, or you can just grow it on your windowsill. Fresh air, plenty of good health and something nice to spice up your dishes. What more could a believer in natural goodness of natural products want?

So it does not matter whether you are in the East or in the West. Get your metabolism working, your auto immune system growing stronger, your lungs healthy with fresh air, your kidneys healthy with leaves and your whole system toned up with Basil tea.

Dry the leaves and sprinkle all over your cooked dishes. Put them in your salt cellar or spice grinder, and enjoy delicious spices. My preferred spice grinder has basil, garlic flakes, rock salt, pepper, ginger flakes, onion flakes, Sage, thyme and Marjoram. The next time round I am going to fill it up with seasoning salts like roasted cumin, rock salt, black salt, basil, ginger flakes, thyme and sage. It is fun experimenting with healthy herbs! I may also try a dried curry powder combination!

So live life king-size and enjoy its natural bounty to the fullest.

Author Bio

Dueep Jyot Singh is a Management and IT Professional who managed to gather Postgraduate qualifications in Management and English and Degrees in Science, French and Education while pursuing different enjoyable career options like being an hospital administrator, IT,SEO and HRD Database Manager/ trainer, movie scriptwriter, theatre artiste and public speaker, lecturer in French, Marketing and Advertising, ex-Editor of Hearts On Fire (now known as Solsctice) Books Missouri USA, advice columnist and cartoonist, publisher and Aviation School trainer, ex- moderator on Medico.in, banker, student councilor ,travelogue writer … among other things! One fine morning, she decided that she had enough of killing herself by Degrees and went back to her first love -- writing. It's more enjoyable! She already has 48 published academic and 14 fiction- in- different- genre books under her belt.

When she is not designing websites or making Graphic design illustrations for clients , she is browsing through old bookshops hunting for treasures, of which she has an enviable collection – including R.L. Stevenson, O.Henry, Dornford Yates, Maurice Walsh, C.N.Williamson, Sapper, Bartimeus and the crown of her collection- Dickens "The Old Curiosity Shop," and so on… Just call her "Renaissance Woman" - collecting herbal remedies, acting like Universal Helping Hand/Agony Aunt, or escaping to her dear mountains for a bit of exploring, collecting herbs and plants, and trekking.

Check out some of the other Health Learning Series books at Amazon.com

Health Learning Series on Amazon

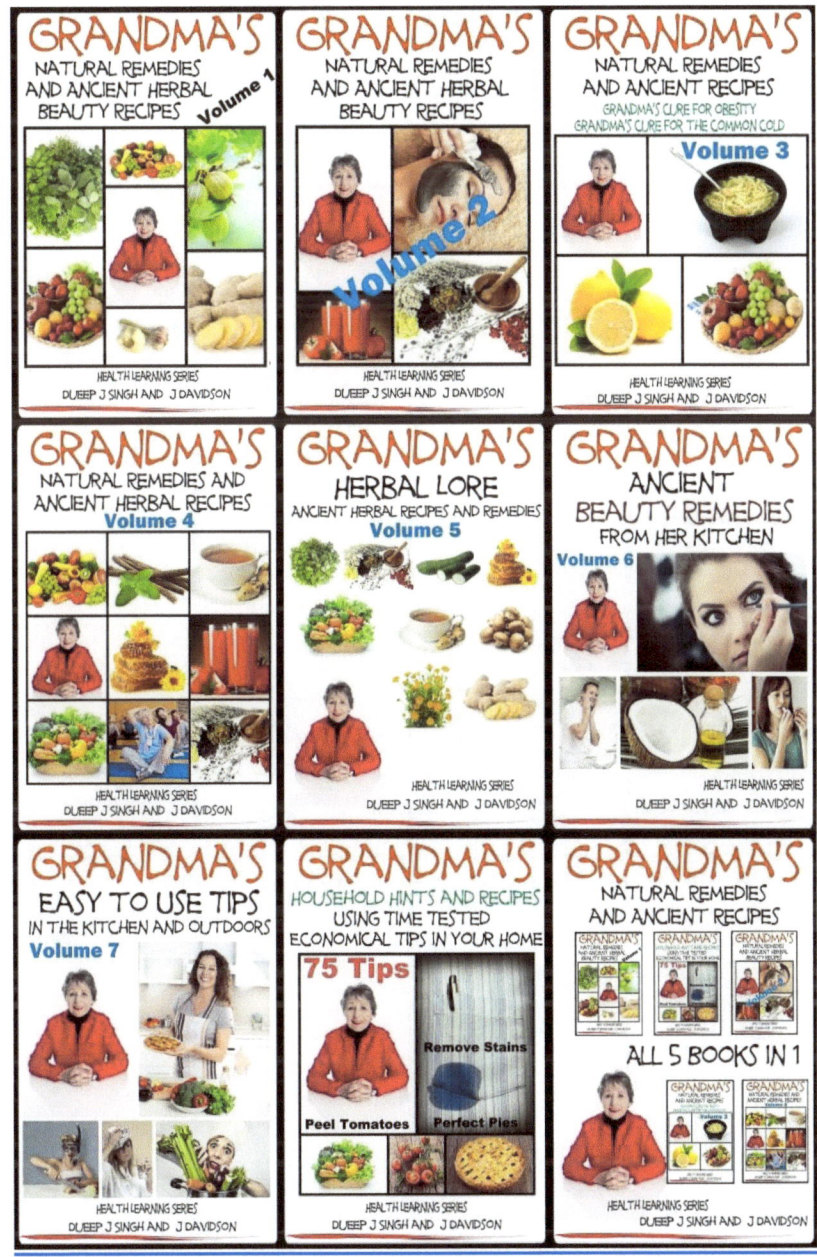

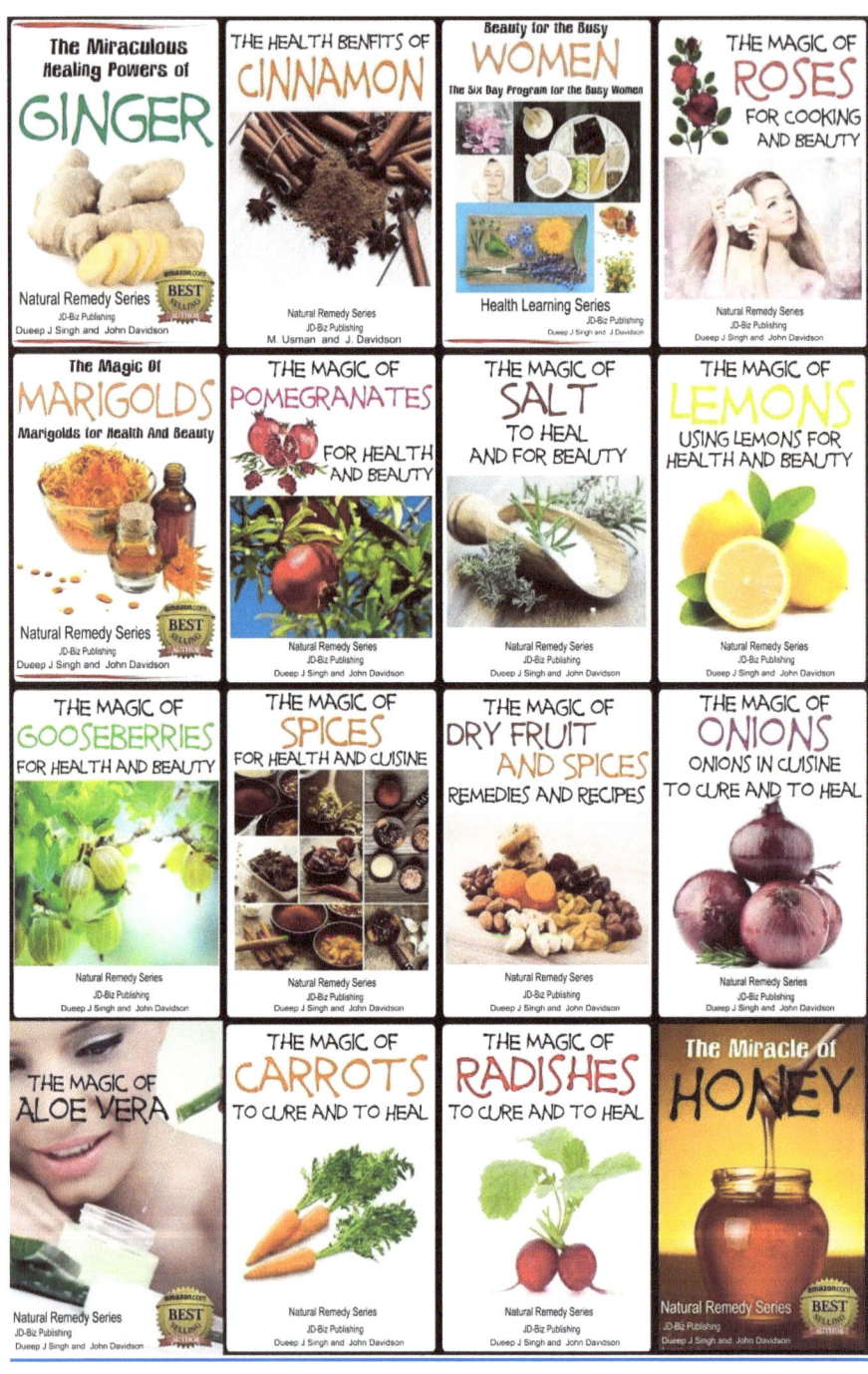

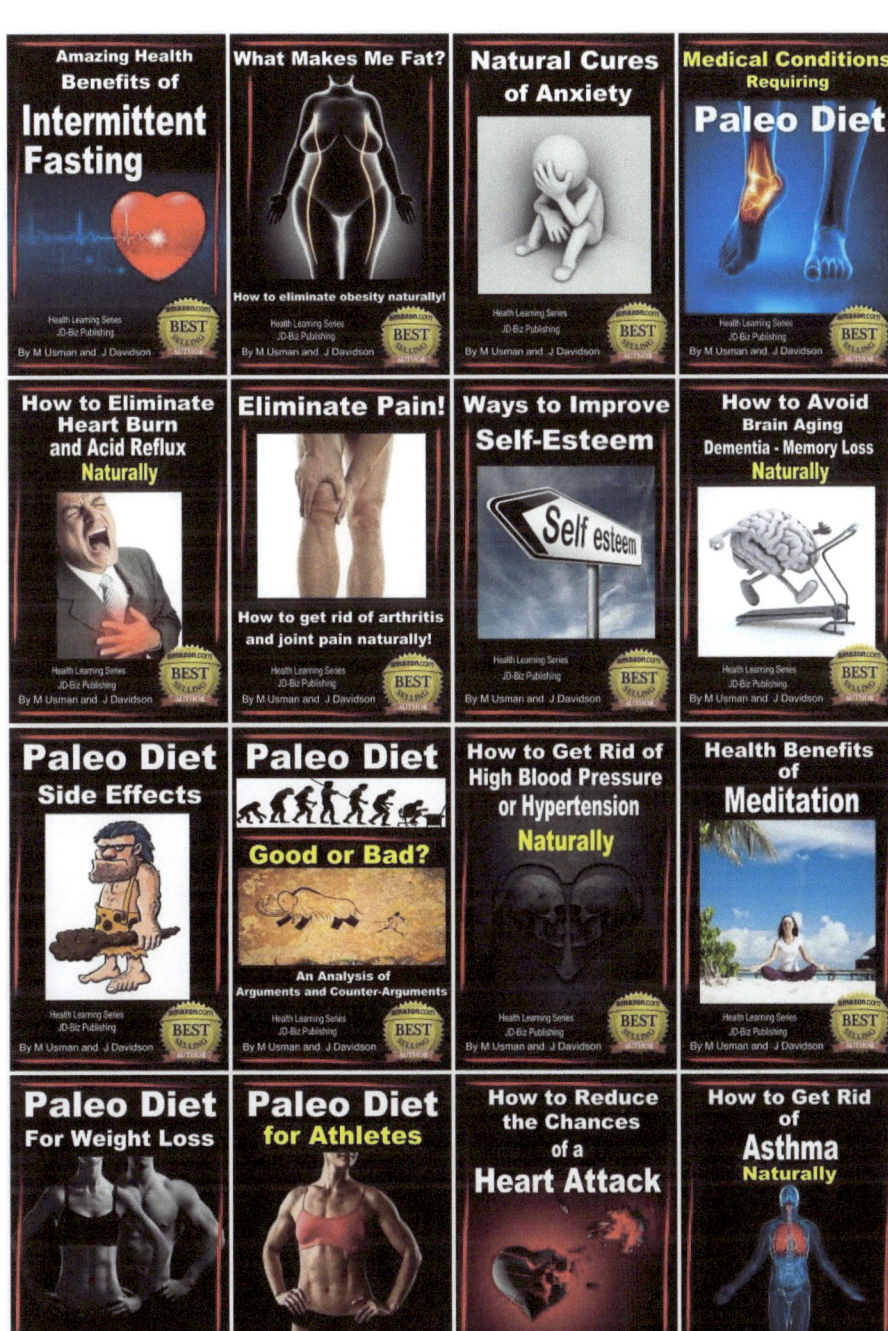

Amazing Animal Books Series

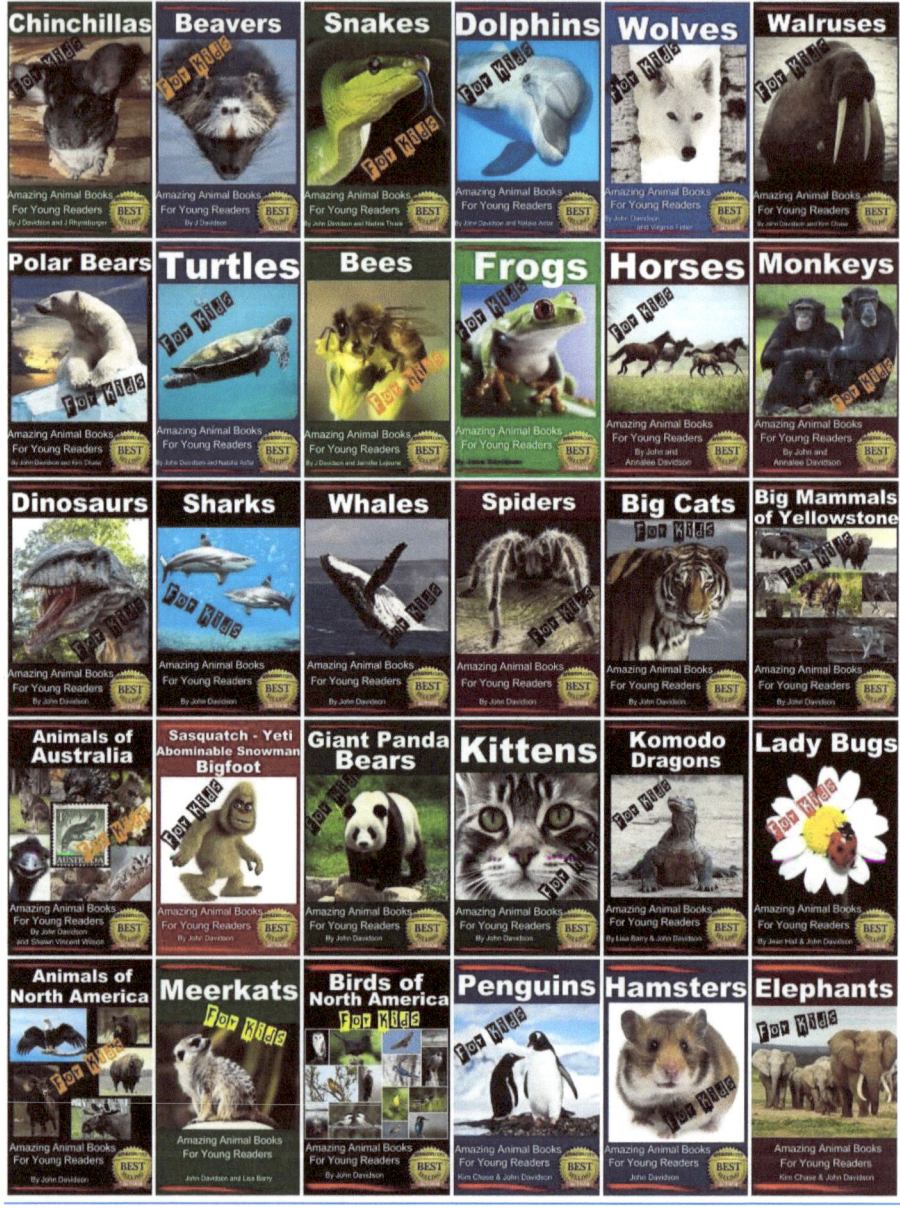

Learn To Draw Series

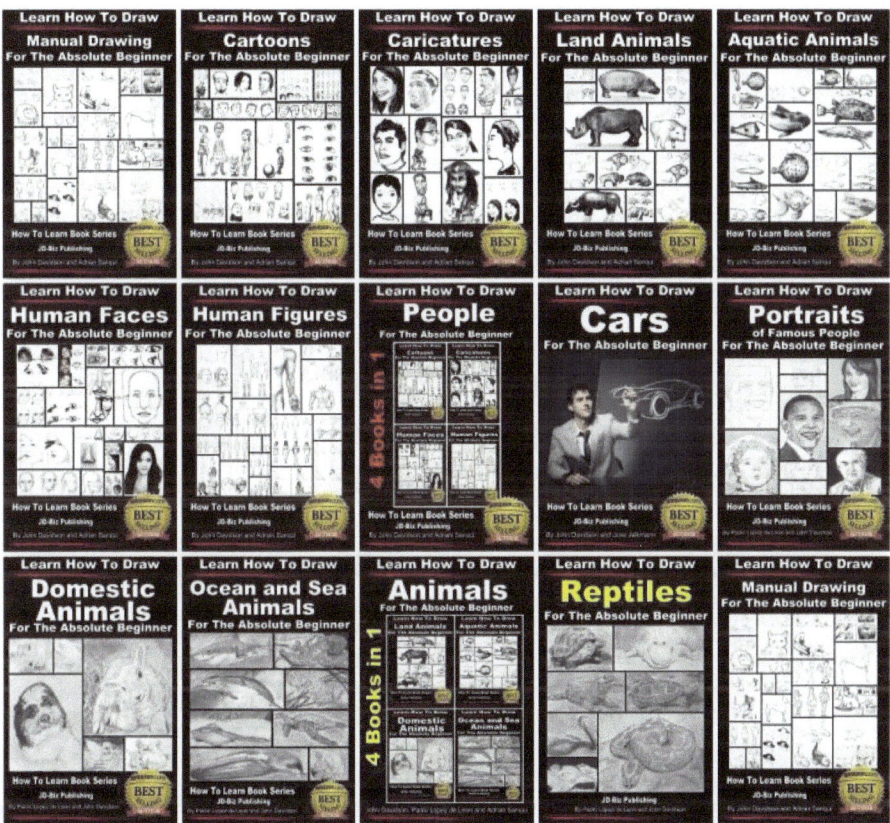

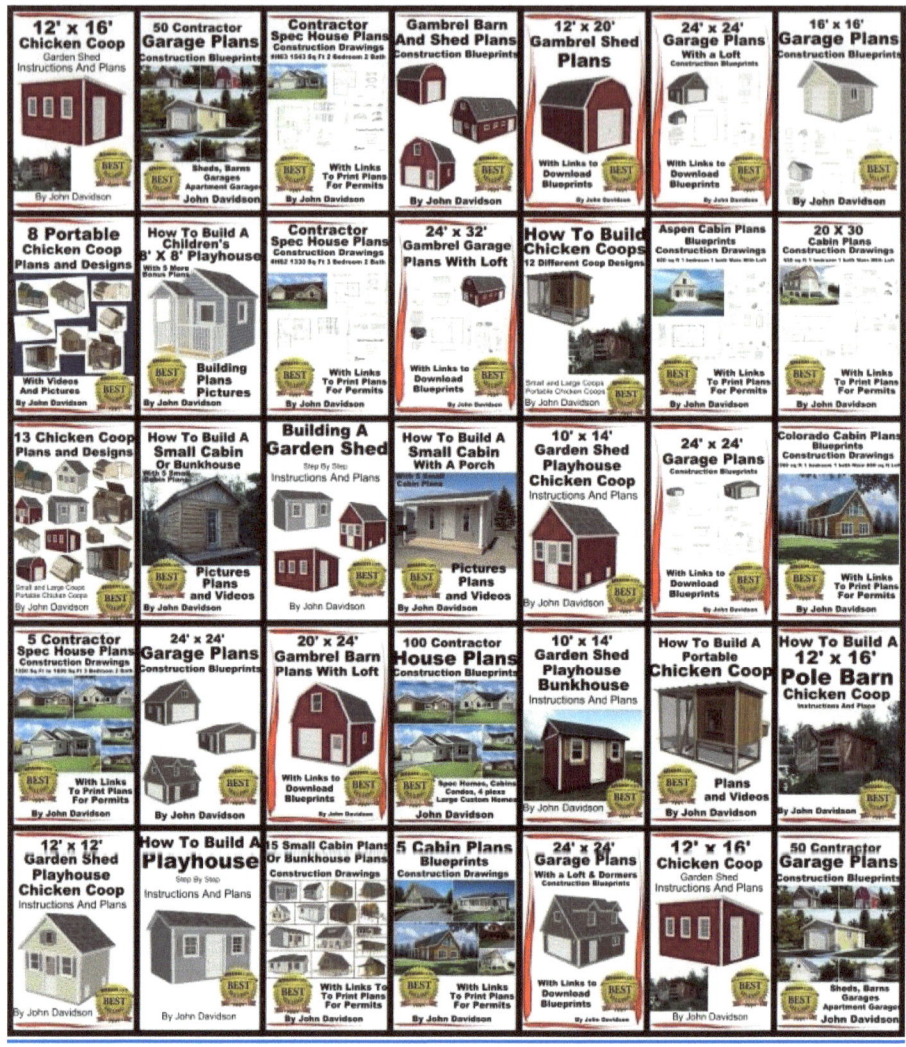

Our books are available at

1. Amazon.com

2. Barnes and Noble

3. Itunes

4. Kobo

5. Smashwords

6. Google Play Books

Download Free Books!

http://MendonCottageBooks.com

Publisher

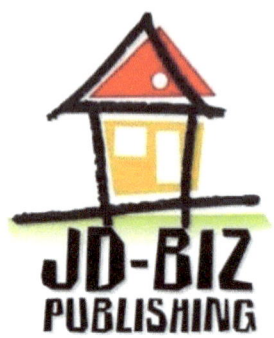

JD-Biz Corp

P O Box 374

Mendon, Utah 84325

http://www.jd-biz.com/

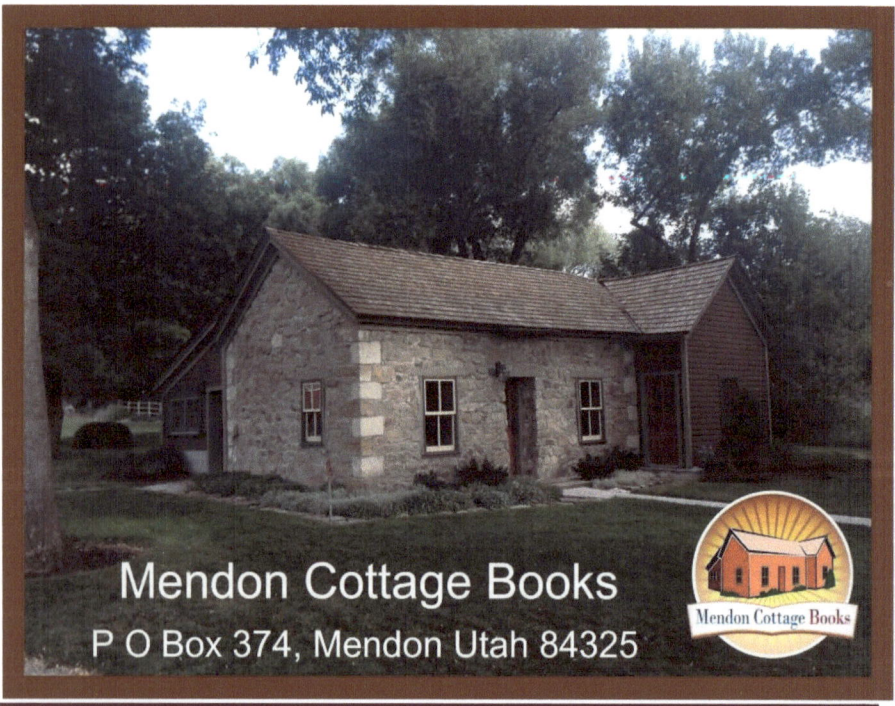

Mendon Cottage Books

P O Box 374, Mendon Utah 84325